Just For You

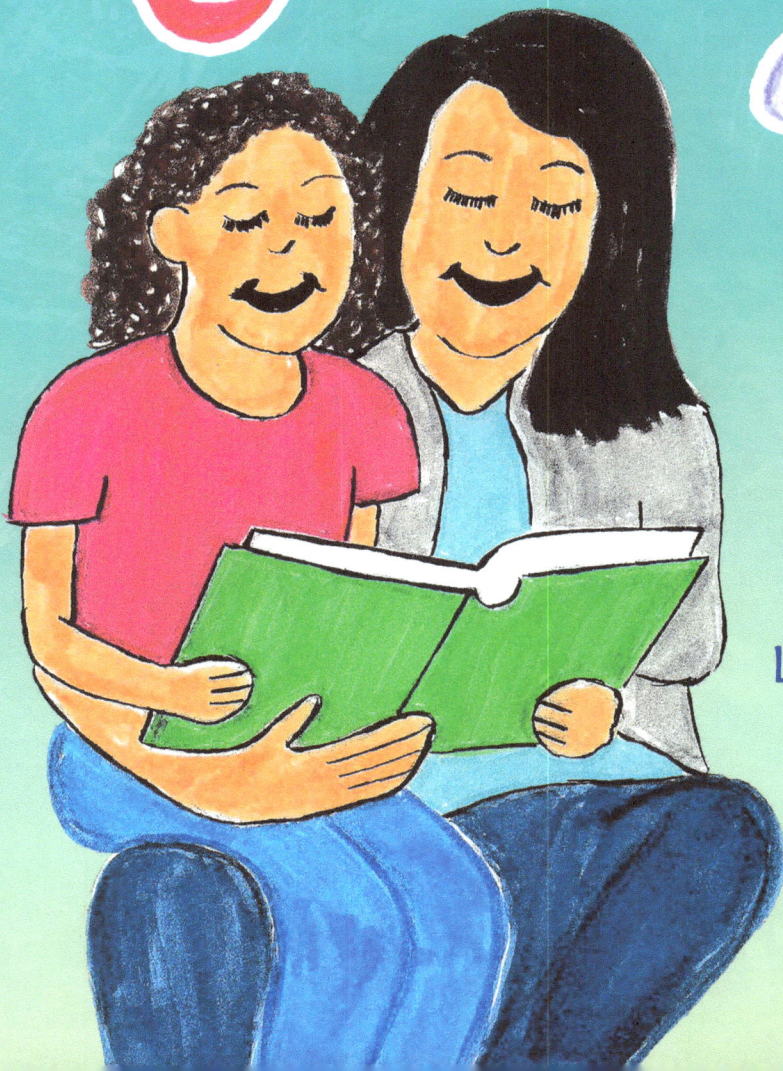

Written by:
LAURIE VINEBERG BUCH

Illustrated by:
SHANNON DEMEO

With Special Illustrations by:
CHARLIE and CASEY BUCH

ISBN:
978-1-63308-460-5 (paperback)
978-1-63308-461-2 (ebook)

Interior Design by *R'tor John D. Maghuyop*
Illustrated by *Shannon DeMeo*
With Special Illustrations by *Charlie and Casey Buch*

CHALFANT ECKERT
PUBLISHING

1028 S Bishop Avenue, Dept. 178
Rolla, MO 65401

Printed in United States of America

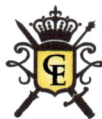

Just For You

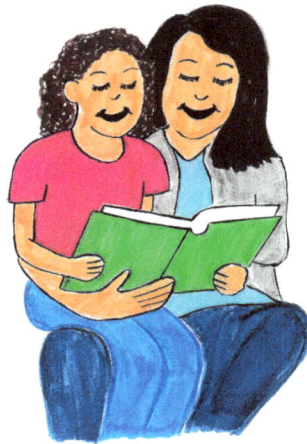

Written by:

LAURIE VINEBERG BUCH

Illustrated by:
SHANNON DEMEO

With Special Illustrations by:
CHARLIE and CASEY BUCH

Acknowledgment

I would like to thank the nurses and doctors at the Montreal Children's Hospital. Dr. Bernard Rosenblatt, Heather Davies and Dr. Kenneth Myers have been extremely helpful and supportive in Charlie's care. The nurses and secretaries at the Montreal Children's Pediatric Day Center have made Charlie's regular treatments as comfortable as they can be. Their care and love for Charlie is immeasurable. This book would not be possible if not for Julie Bergeron. Julie, thank you for bringing my book to life.

I would like to thank my family and friends. Over the years you have all shown tremendous support for our family. Growing up, my parents instilled the value of family and putting loved ones first, my sister and I have embraced this value in good times and rough patches. Thank you for the morning greetings, the smoothies, the manicures and the candy surprises. Charlie is lucky to have 4 grandparents who love her dearly and many aunts, uncles and cousins who make her feel special.

To Mark, my best friend, I love you and thank you for pushing me to be better than I think I am. To my girls. Three beautiful girls that make me feel like the luckiest mom. Cameron, only a baby but still my trooper, always there to give me a smile when I desperately need one. Casey, my light, my Jellybean the energy in the house, your enthusiasm and caring nature keeps me motivated to always be on the top of my game. Charlie, my peanut, my brave soul, the heart of the family. You amaze me, you don't let your epilepsy stop you from enjoying life and everyone looks up to you, especially me.

My wish is that a cure for epilepsy is found, I thank all medical professionals who are dedicated to finding a cure for this condition.

Dear Charlie,

This book was made to answer some questions you have.

You are 4 now, and Mummy and Daddy feel you are big enough to learn about something you have had since you were a baby.

It is just a small part of who you are, but you are old enough to learn about it and know the answers to all of your questions.

Dear Charlie,

This book was made to answer some questions you have. You are 4 now and Mummy and Daddy feel you are big enough to learn about something you have had since you were a baby. It is just a small part of who you are but you are old enough to learn about it and know the answers to all of your questions. Love, Mummy & Daddy

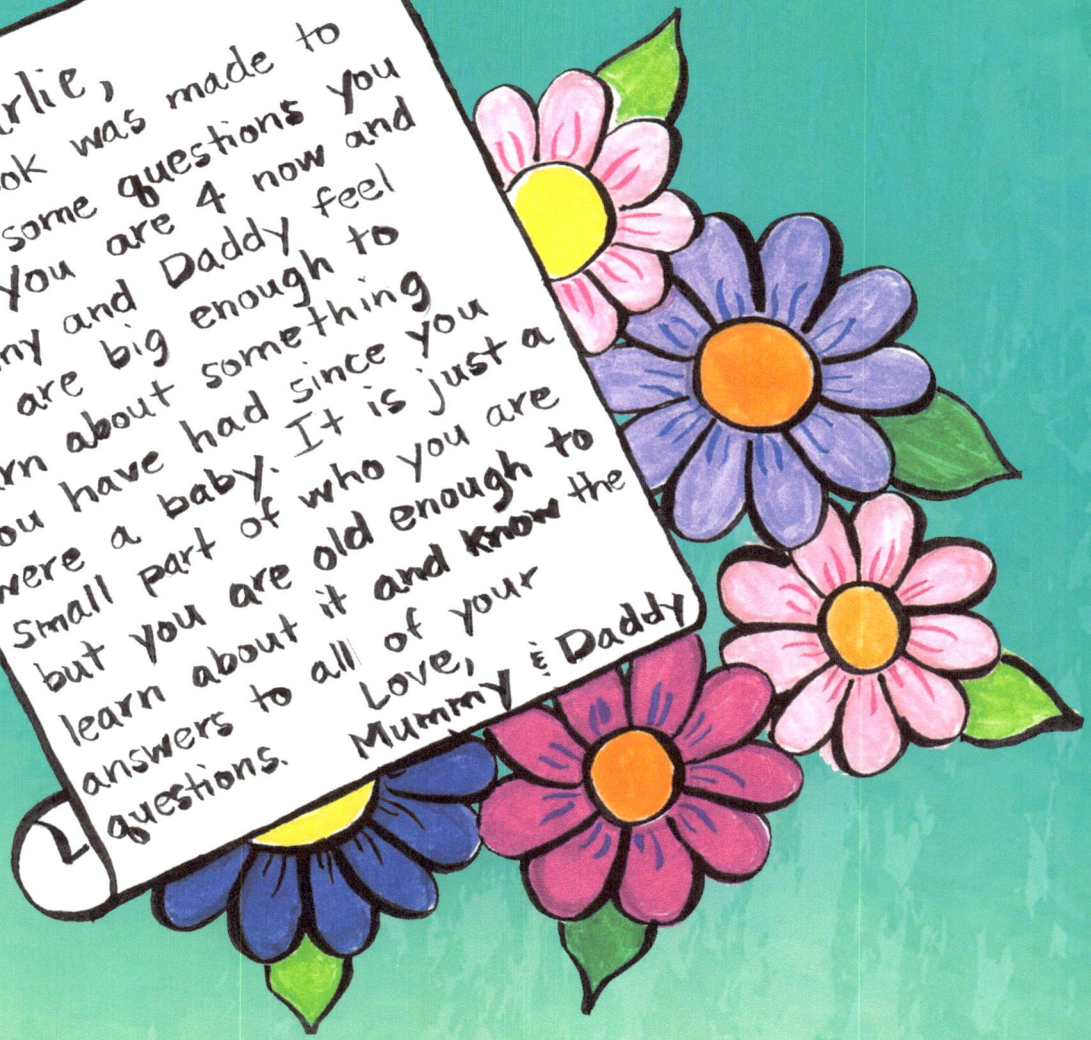

You have something called epilepsy.

Epilepsy means sometimes
your hand shakes and tingles,
and you can't stop it.

These shakes and tingles
are called seizures.

Lots and lots of people have epilepsy,
the same way lots of people wear
glasses like Mummy.

One important thing to remember
is if you can stop your hand from
shaking, then it is not a seizure.

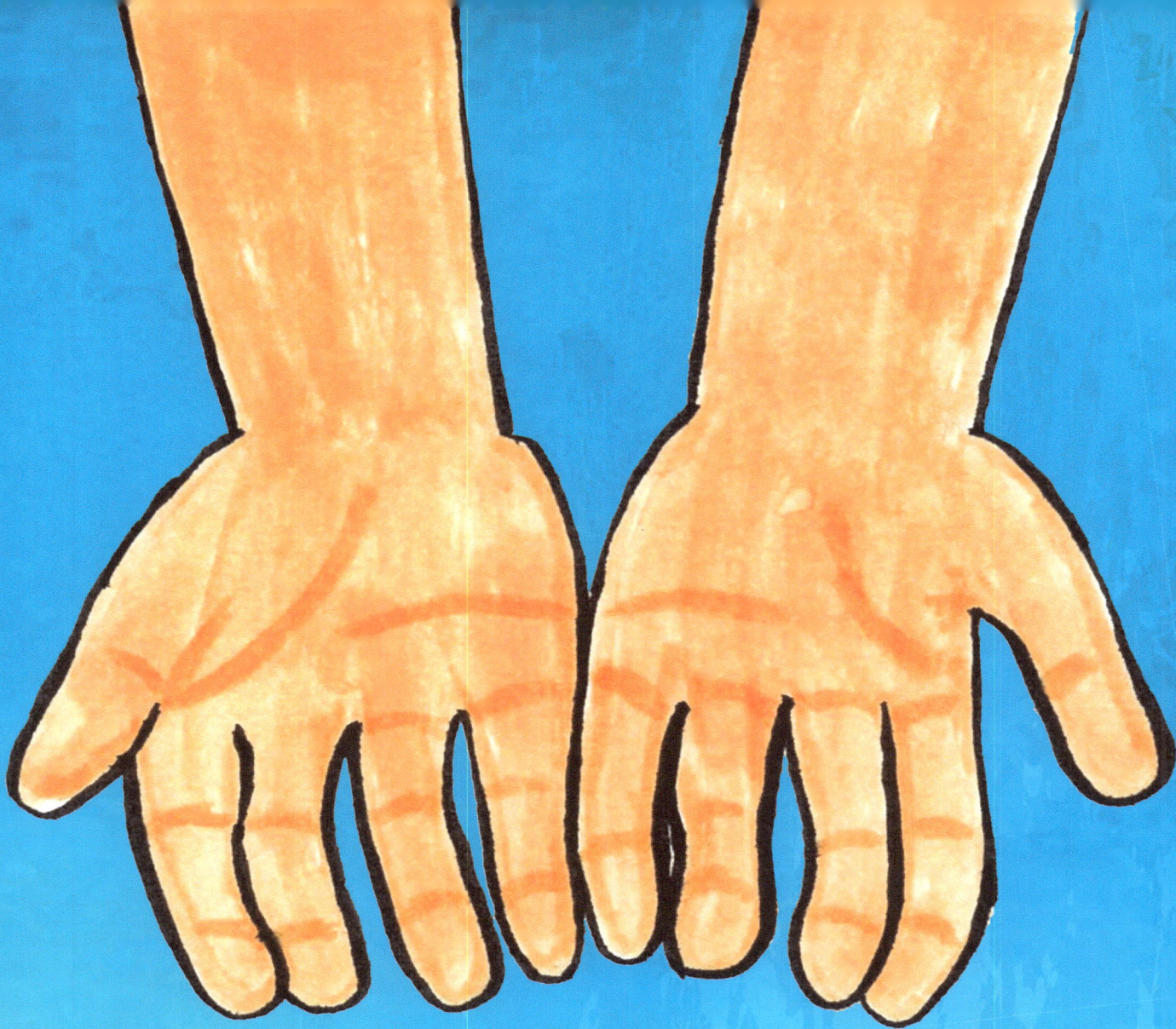

You take medicine called Frisium, Topomax and Fycompa to help prevent a seizure - that means to stop it from happening.

People all over the world take medicine everyday for lots of reasons.

Kids take medicine for epilepsy, just like you. They also take medicine everyday for other reasons.

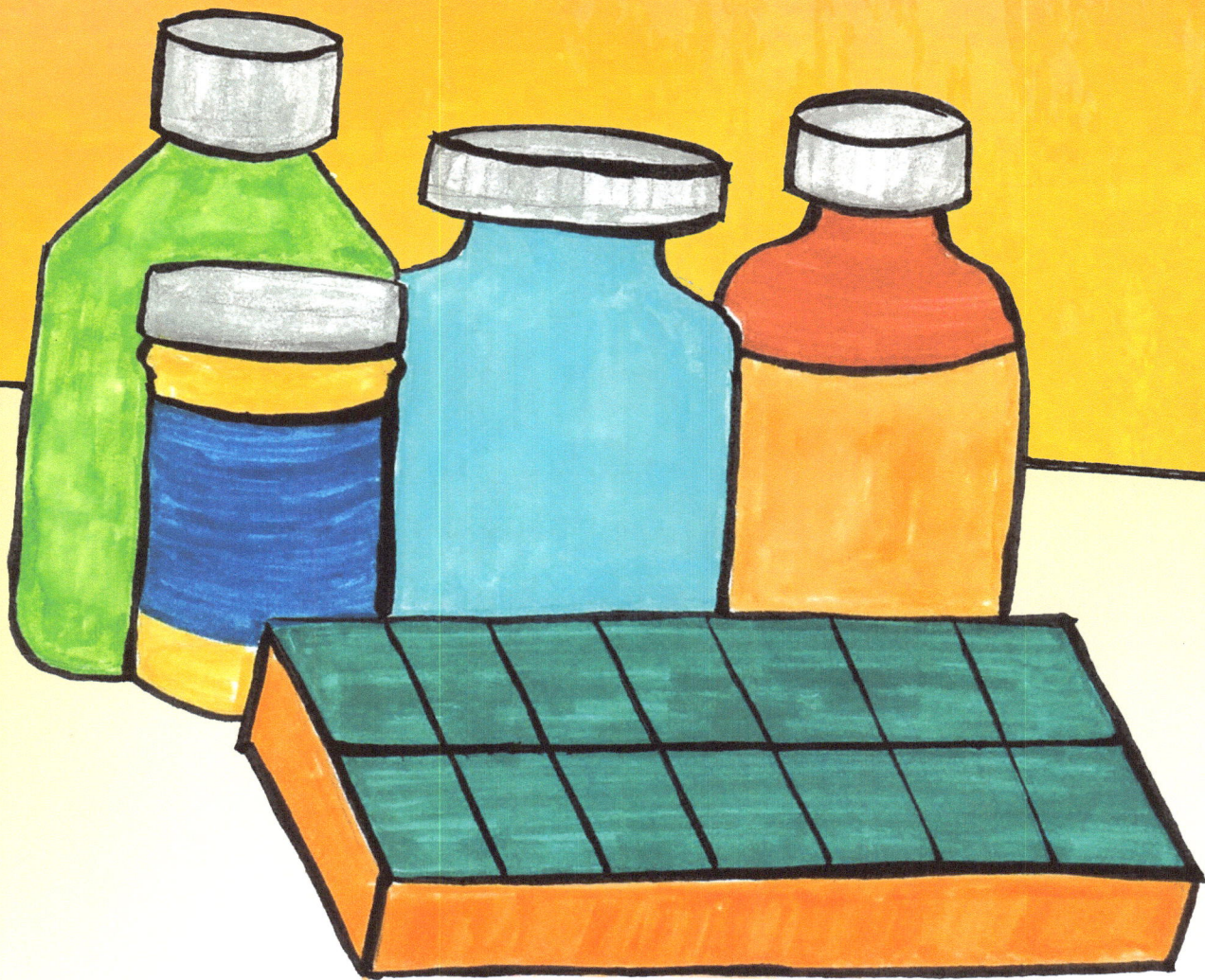

Bubbie takes medicine to keep her
body healthy. Noah and Kyle take
their puffs so they can breathe better.
They are just like you!

When people have headaches
or fever they take Tylenol and Advil.
These are medicines you take only
when you feel yucky or have
your treatments.

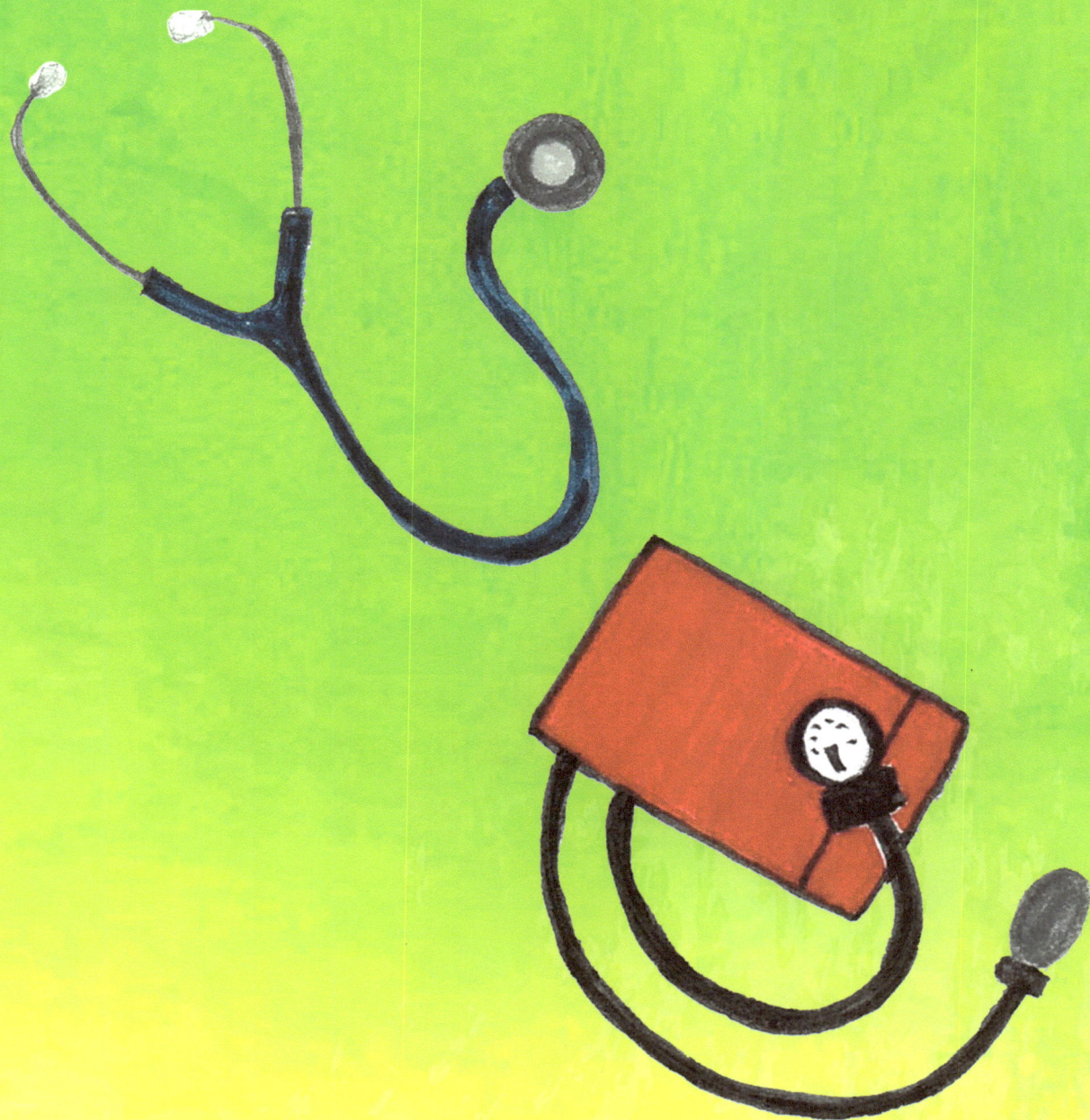

Everyone goes to the doctor - it's part of life! Daddy is a doctor and he sees people everyday for many reasons.

You have two doctors. Dr. Treherne is your regular doctor. We go to him for yearly check ups and if you have a really bad cough or cold. Presely and Callie go see Dr. Treherne, too!

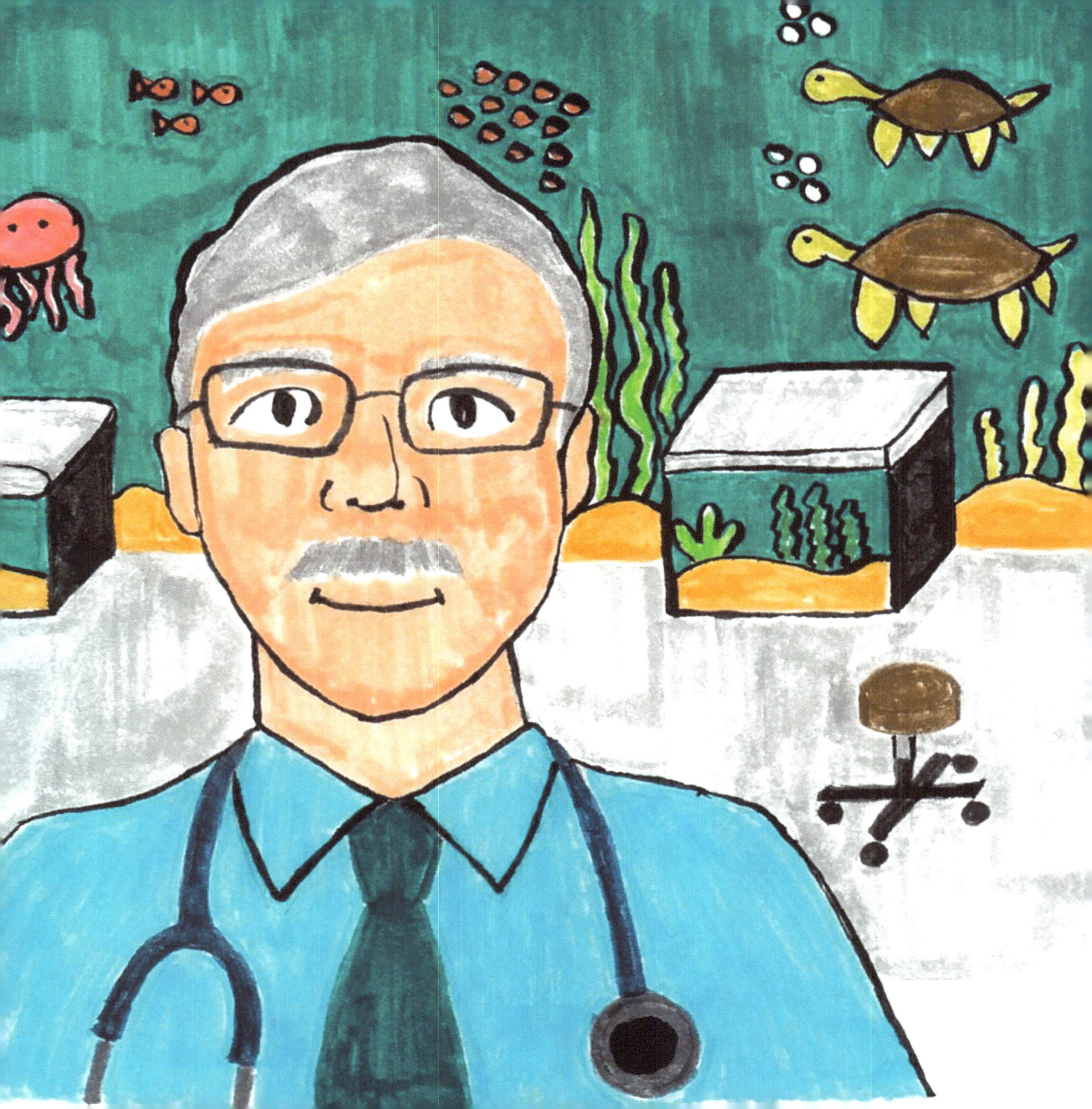

Dr. Myers is the doctor we go to for epilepsy.

He is an expert and he helps us make sure your hand shakes less. He is sometimes funny, too!

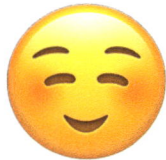

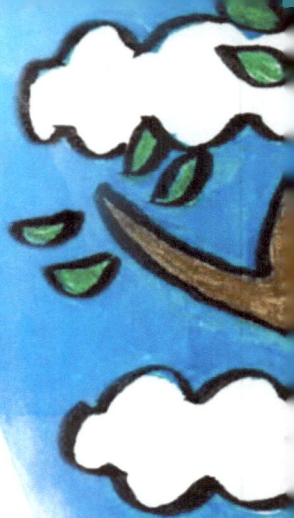

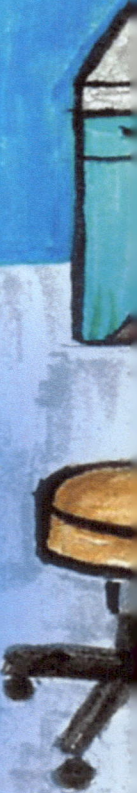

☺️

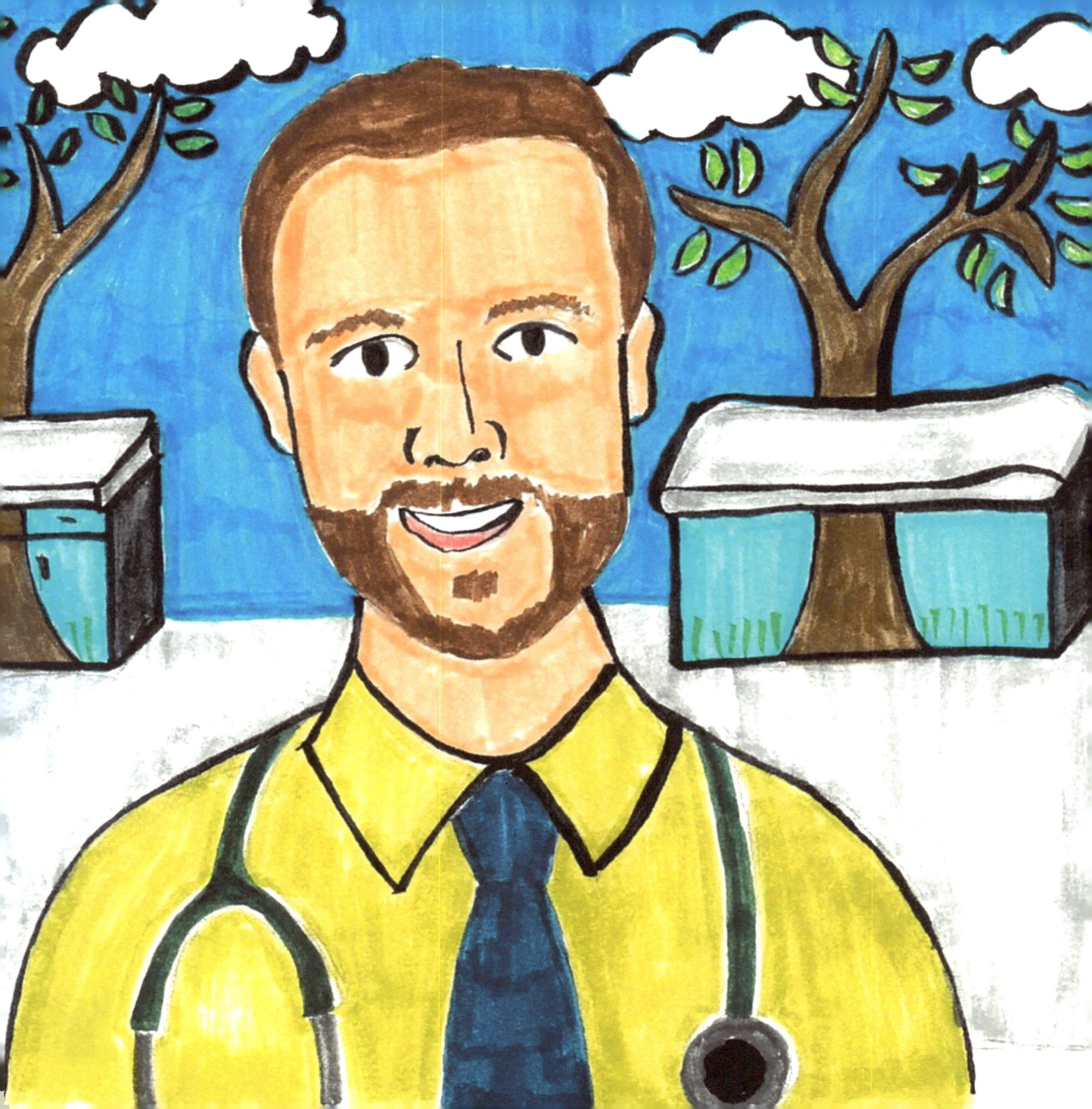

Every month we go see Anne and
the other nurses for your treatment.
Your treatments also help control
your tingling and shaking.

We know it isn't the most fun
BUT we also get to hang out, play
games, see princesses and watch
lots of movies.

You are so amazing during your
treatments Mummy and Daddy are
SOOOOO proud of you!

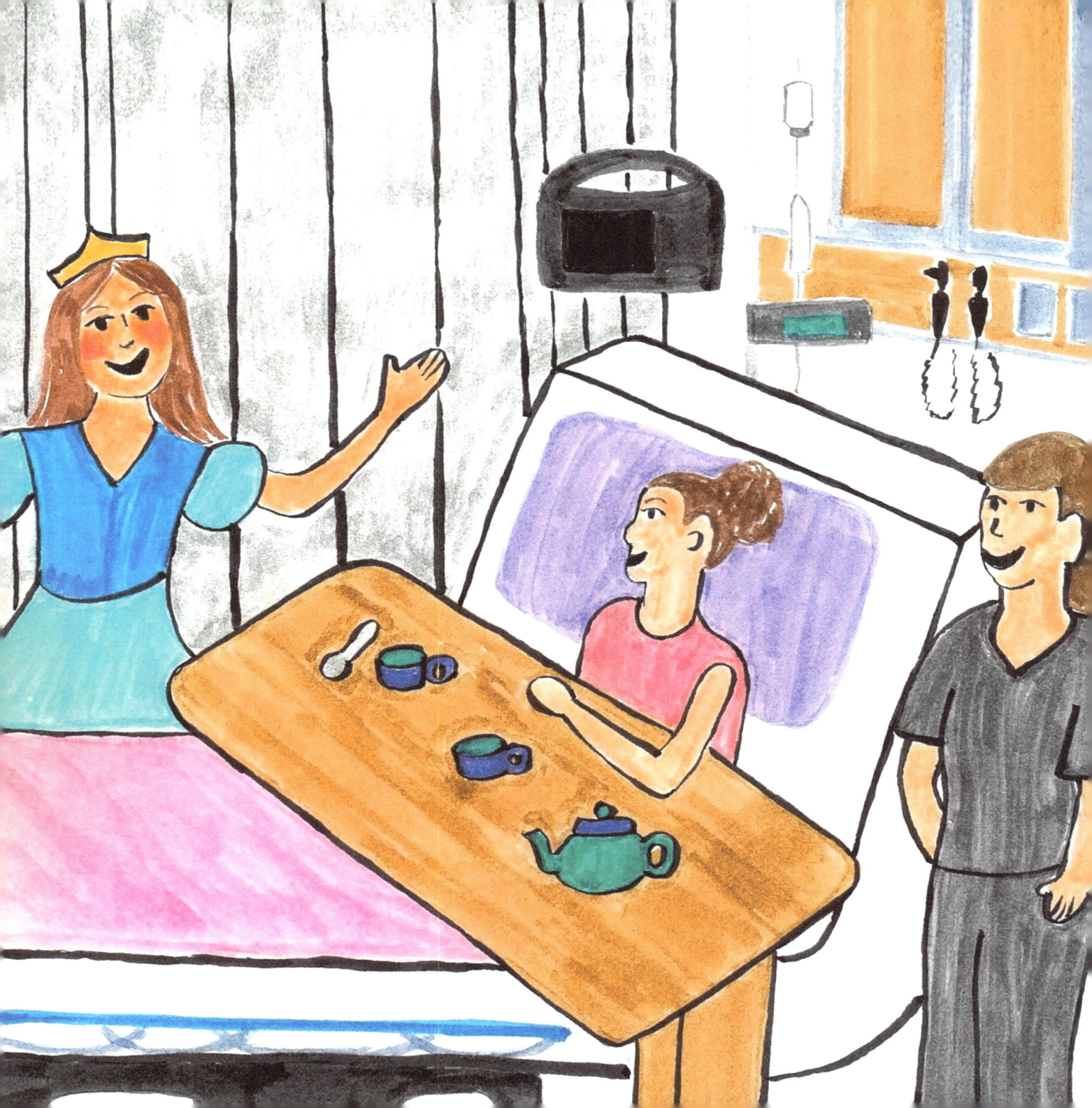

Sometimes you need to go to the hospital for an EEG. An EEG is a crown that you have to wear and it has lots of rainbow wires.

This is a recording of all the things happening in your brain. It is sooo cool that we can have a story of what is going on in your brain. Many adults and children do EEGs and even Mummy did one when she was a kid

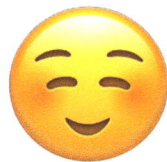

☺️

The good thing about the EEG is that they DON'T HURT and you get to see all the rainbow wires.

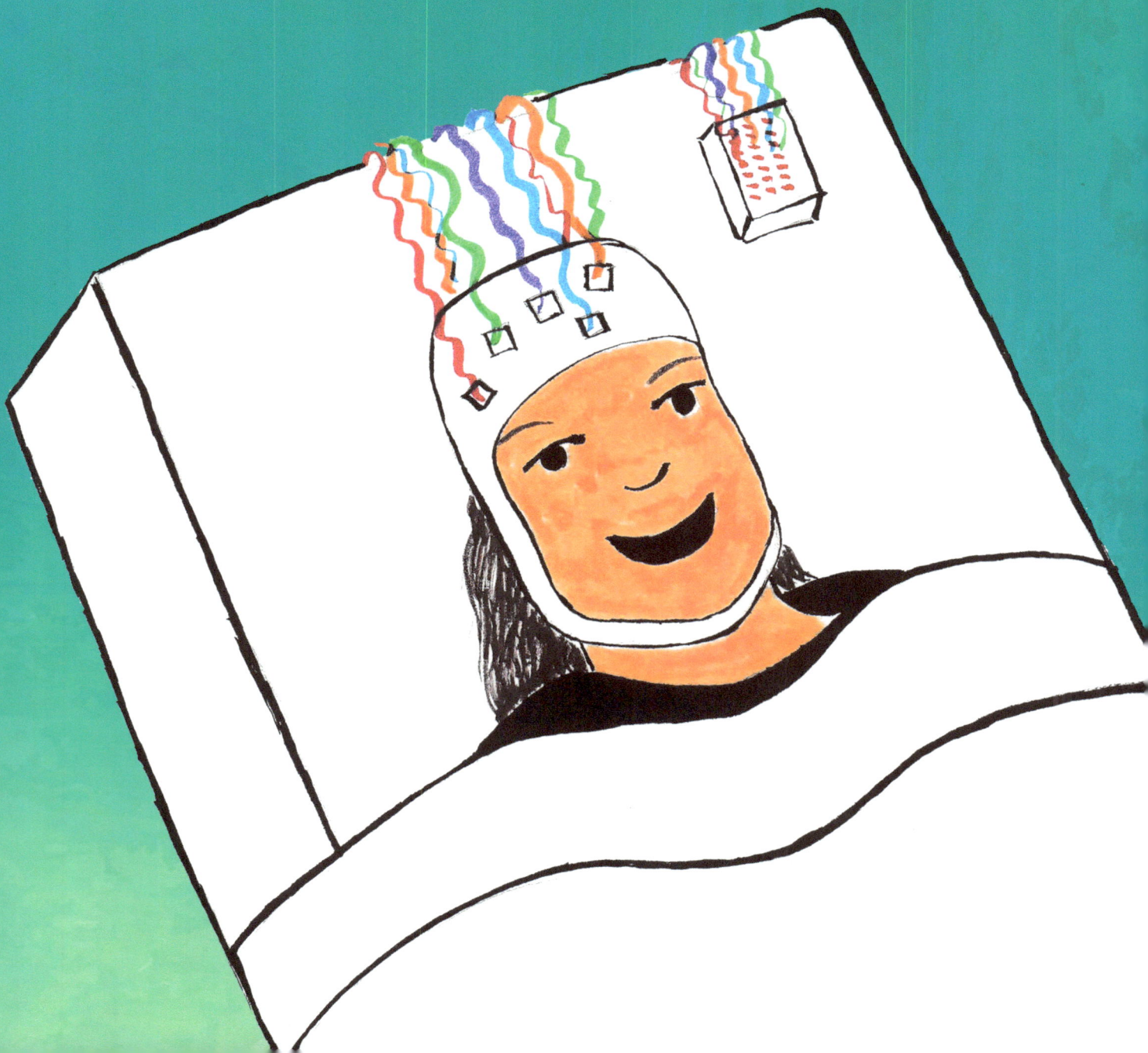

We hope this book has answered some of your questions.

Here are some important things to remember:

1. You are a healthy and brave girl!

2. You have epilepsy and that means sometimes your hand shakes and tingles.

3. The medicine you take and the hospital visits help control the shaking and tingling.

4. People all over the world take medicine just like you.

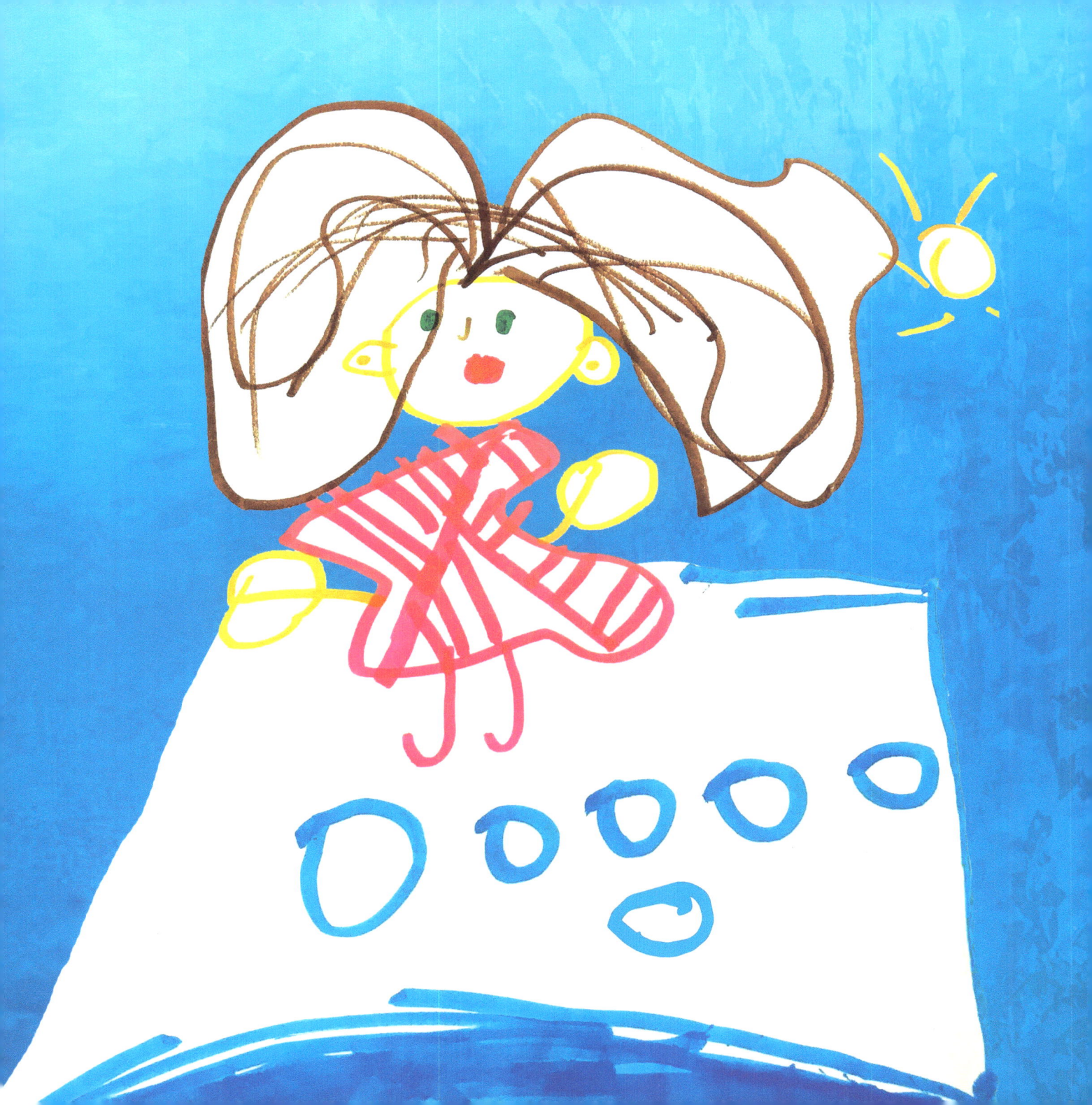

MOST OF ALL, REMEMBER YOU ARE
AN AMAZING AND SPECIAL GIRL

BECAUSE YOU ARE KIND, FUNNY,
SILLY, SMART, BRAVE, GENEROUS,

STRONG AND ABOVE ALL THE
BEST THING IN THE WHOLE
WIDE WORLD!!

WE LOVE YOU!!!

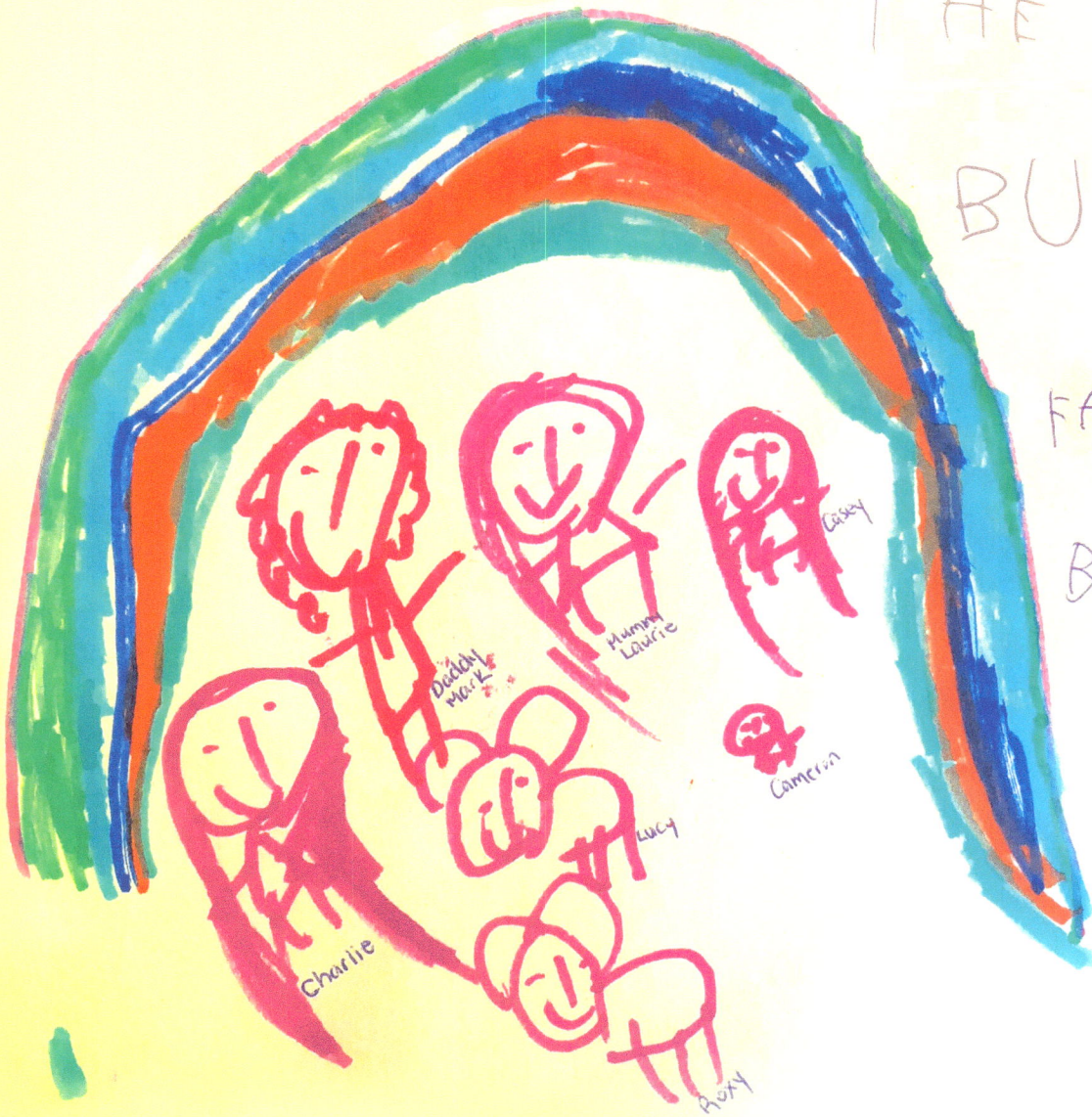

"Thank you Michael Flatley,
Shannon DeMeo from Books that
Heal for the published book.
I hope all the other kids with
epilepsy feel better.
Love Charlie."

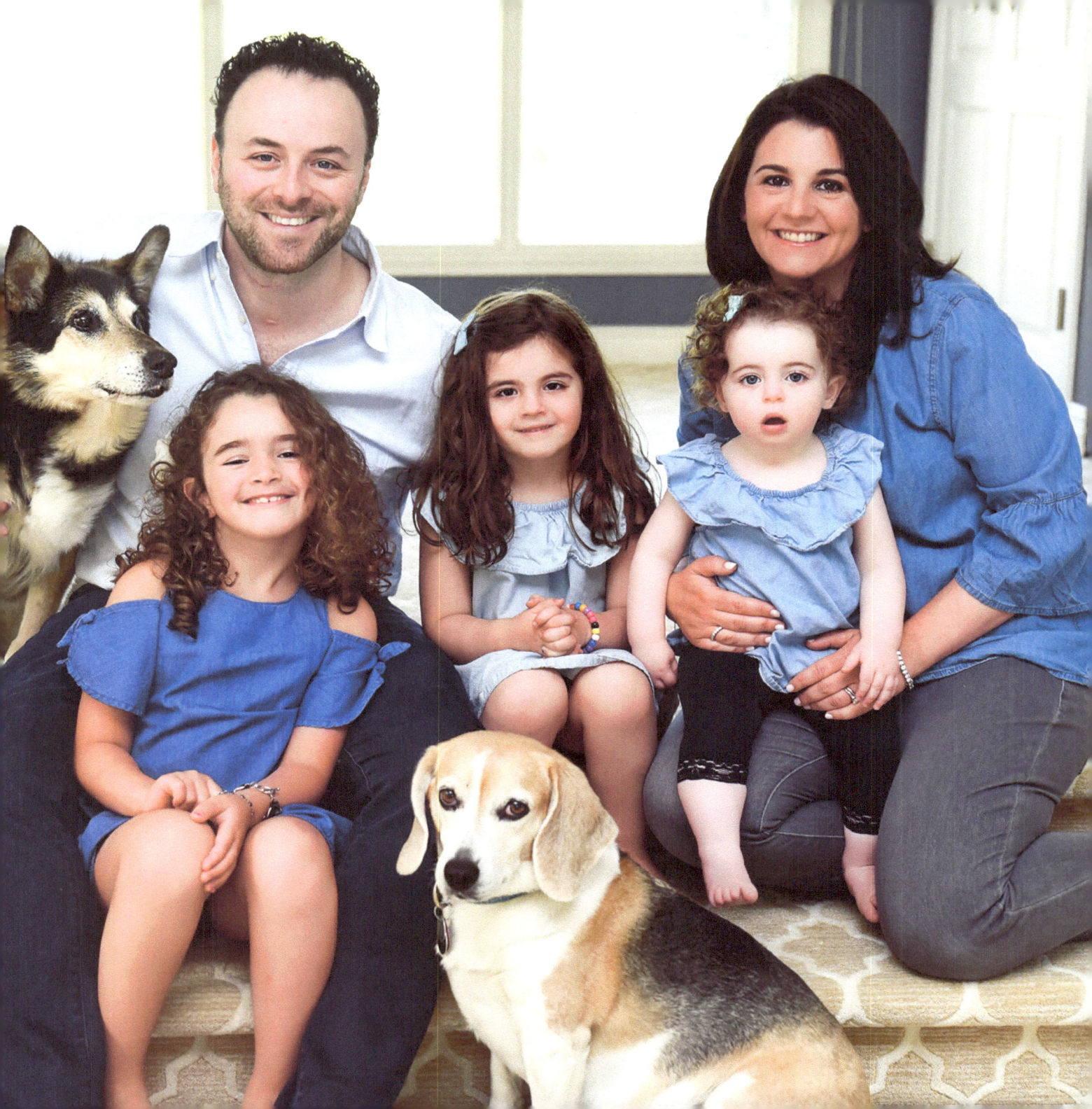